TABLE OF CONTENTMENT

TABLE OF CONTENTMENT

MOTIVATION

WHAT'S YOURS?

To achieve something, you need to have a vision. An end goal so to speak. Some say "Focus on the journey, not the destination". For us who stand to lose a few pounds, the quicker we arrive at the destination, the better.

What are your reasons for losing weight?

01   **Health**

02   **Cosmetic**

03   **Work**

04   **Relationship**

VITAL STATS

LET'S GET IT OVER WITH

I hate this part. Writing it down.
Setting it in stone, where anybody can read it and laugh at my BMI.
However, to achieve results, you need empirical data. BEFORE and AFTER.
It is the only way to measure if your method works or not.
So get that measuring tape out and record this down.

DATE

NAME

SEX
Male / Female / It's complicated

WEIGHT
kg / lbs

HEIGHT
cm / ft

WAIST
cm / inch

ASS
cm / inch

BMI

AGE
years young

Category BMI range - kg/m2
Severe Thinness < 16
Moderate Thinness 16 - 17
Mild Thinness 17 - 18.5
Normal 18.5 - 25
Overweight 25 - 30
Obese Class I 30 - 35
Obese Class II 35 - 40
Obese Class III > 40

VITAL STATS
SUBSEQUENT ATTEMPTS

This is not a misprint.
Hopefully the values are lowered and you see some improvement.
Otherwise, abandon your current method and try something else!

DATE

WEIGHT kg / lbs

HEIGHT cm / ft

WAIST cm / inch

ASS cm / inch

BMI

AGE years young

Category BMI range - kg/m2
Severe Thinness < 16
Moderate Thinness 16 - 17
Mild Thinness 17 - 18.5
Normal 18.5 - 25
Overweight 25 - 30
Obese Class I 30 - 35
Obese Class II 35 - 40
Obese Class III > 40

VITAL STATS

SUBSEQUENT ATTEMPTS

This is not a misprint.
Hopefully the values are lowered and you see some improvement.
Otherwise, abandon your current method and try something else!

DATE

WEIGHT kg / lbs

HEIGHT cm / ft

WAIST cm / inch

ASS cm / inch

BMI

AGE years young

Category BMI range - kg/m2
Severe Thinness < 16
Moderate Thinness 16 - 17
Mild Thinness 17 - 18.5
Normal 18.5 - 25
Overweight 25 - 30
Obese Class I 30 - 35
Obese Class II 35 - 40
Obese Class III > 40

MY BODY

Current picture
Version 1.0

Future picture
Version 2.0

a body to die for

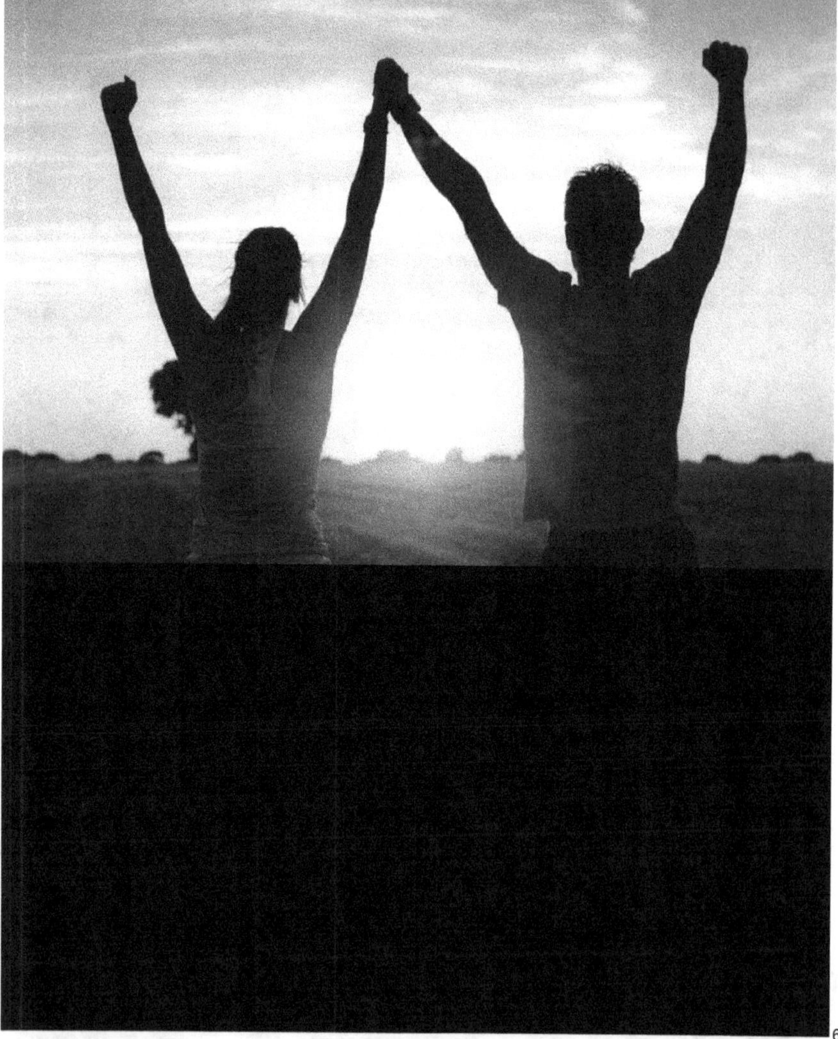

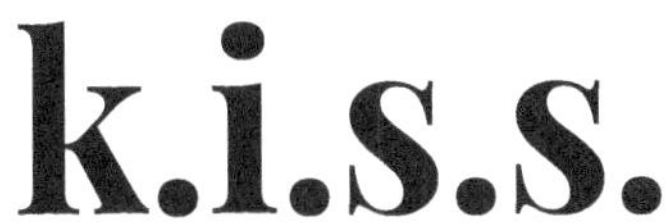

keep it simple sally

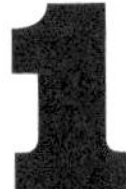

1 what you eat

what you shovel into your mouth matters

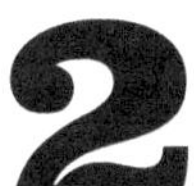

2 when you eat

Naturally you digest better in the day
compared to night
Follow the sun. Metabolism at its peak from
10am to 2pm

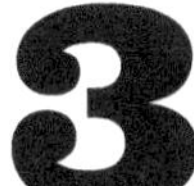

3 what you do

Our bodies are not designed to be
sedentary
Move as much as you can.

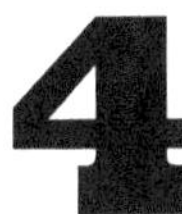

4 what you add-on

Supplement what you lack

D.I.E...T

Imagine for a moment that you were given a car. It is free. It gets you around places. All you have to do is maintain it. There are no options to replace the car when it breaks down.

How would you take care of this car? Would you pour cheap or processed fuel into the car? Can the car perform optimally if it rarely goes over 50mph? When you start the car in the morning, do you immediately force it to speed? Would you schedule bi annual service in the garage to ensure the car's long life?

Treat your body as if it were this car. Feed it only wholesome, non processed fuel. Lubricant for the car, and water for you, is important. When the car is clean, and properly maintained, it will serve you for many years to come.

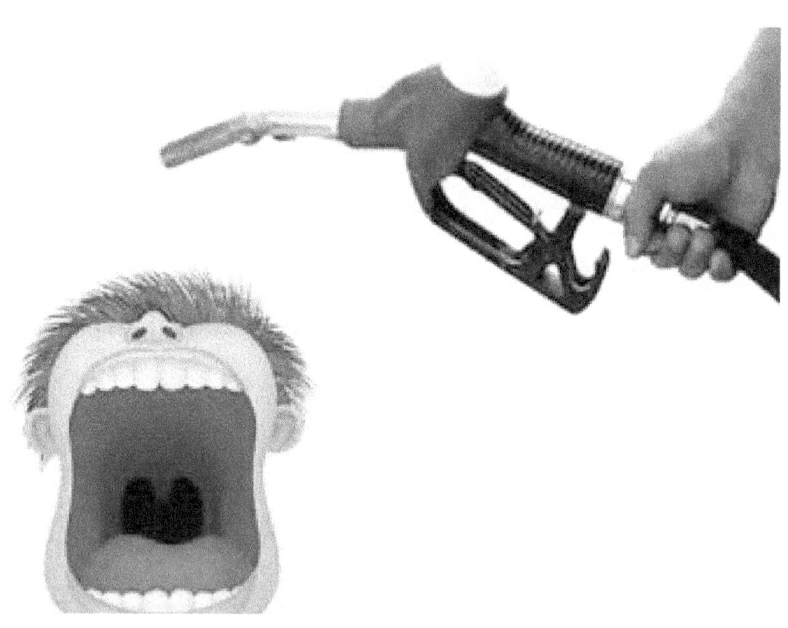

Good fuel   Bad fuel

Date

Date

Date

Date

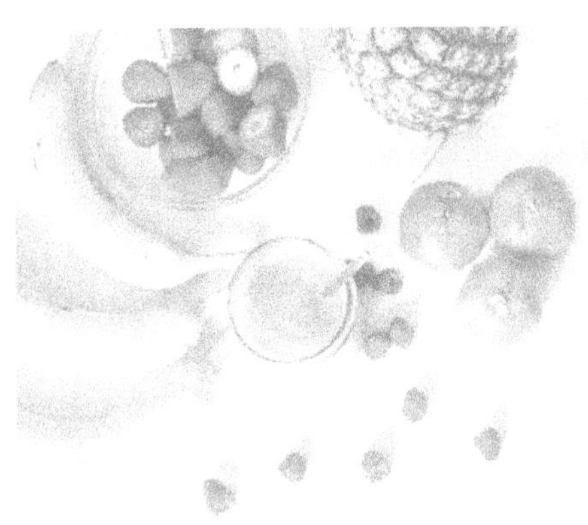

Good fuel   Bad fuel

Date

Date

Date

Date

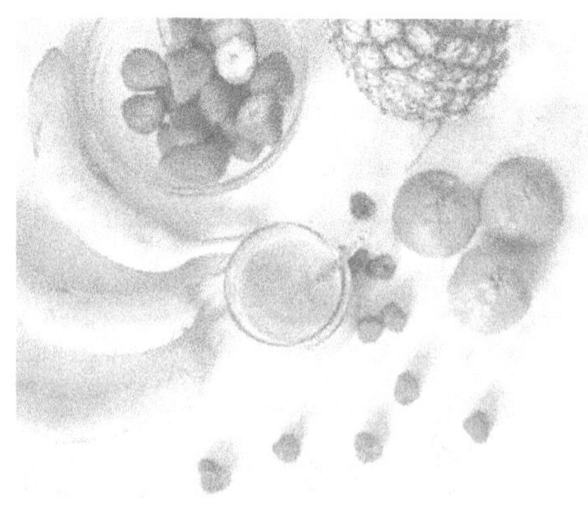

Good fuel   Bad fuel

Date

Date

Date

Date

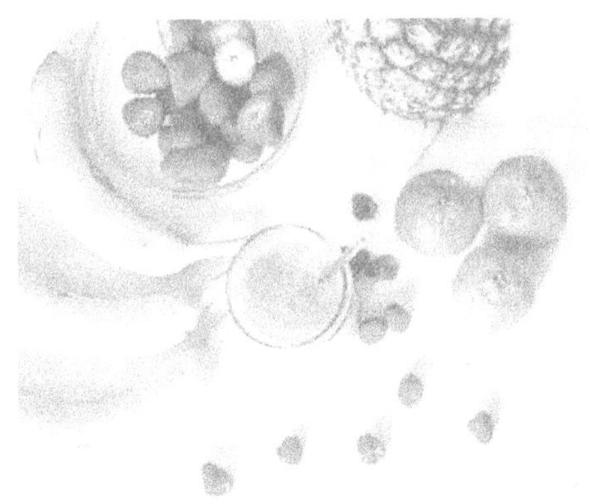

Date

Date

Date

Date

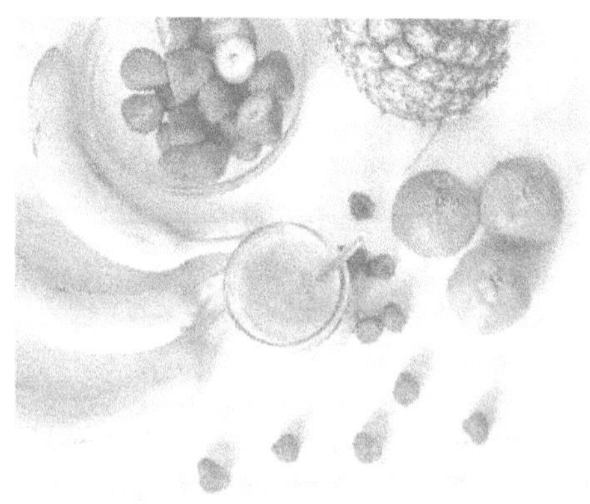

TERMINAL

The quickest way to stop unhealthy eating so that you would lose weight is to scare yourself silly.

Most of us are hypochondriacs to a certain degree. Remember that extra mole you found near your navel? Was that a lump? Are my thyroids inflamed? Why do I have that shoulder ache? Am I experiencing heart palpitations?

Use these symptoms and imagine you have an incurable disease, but the symptoms might dissipate if you start eating healthy, right here, right now. It's your life at stake, but if you continue unhealthy eating habits, <insert terminal disease here> will be imminent.

Prevention is better than cure. There is no "I'll start next year", or "After this bagel" excuse. Next year might already be too late and your condition is irreversible.

* Disclaimer: if you do experience such symptoms long term, please consult the advice of a medical practitioner.

If I don't lose weight, my greatest fear is....

If I don't lose weight, my greatest fear is.....

If I don't lose weight, my greatest fear is.....

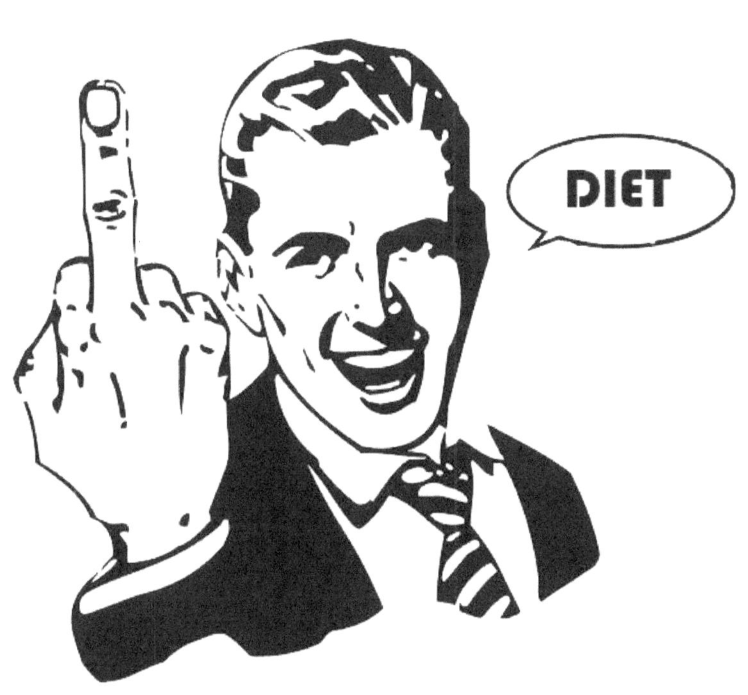
DIET

D.I.E...T

keto

paleo

BURNING FAT FOR FUEL INSTEAD OF
YOUR BODY'S GO-TO ENERGY
SOURCE: CARBS. TO DO THIS, YOU
NEED TO EAT A WHOLE LOT OF FAT.

WHAT YOU CAN EAT
MEATS - FISH, BEEF, LAMB,
POULTRY, EGGS,
LEAFY GREENS - SPINACH, KALE.
ABOVE GROUND VEGETABLES -
BROCCOLI, CAULIFLOWER
HIGH FAT DAIRY - HARD CHEESES,
HIGH FAT CREAM, BUTTER.
NUTS AND SEEDS - MACADAMIAS,
WALNUTS, SUNFLOWER SEEDS.
AVOCADO AND BERRIES -
RASPBERRIES, BLACKBERRIES, AND
OTHER LOW GLYCEMIC IMPACT
BERRIES
SWEETENERS - STEVIA, ERYTHRITOL,
MONK FRUIT, AND OTHER LOW-
CARB SWEETENERS >
OTHER FATS - COCONUT OIL, HIGH-
FAT SALAD DRESSING, SATURATED
FATS, ETC.

BAN LIST
GRAINS - WHEAT, CORN, RICE,
CEREAL, ETC.
SUGAR - HONEY, AGAVE, MAPLE
SYRUP, ETC.
FRUIT - APPLES, BANANAS,
ORANGES, ETC.
TUBERS - POTATO, YAMS, ETC.

THE PALEO DIET, SOMETIMES
REFERRED TO AS "THE CAVEMAN DIET,"
IS BASED ON THE PRINCIPLE THAT
EATING FOODS THAT WERE AVAILABLE
TO EARLY HUMANS WILL PROMOTE
OPTIMAL HEALTH.

WHAT YOU CAN EAT
MEAT AND FISH
EGGS
NUTS AND SEEDS
FRUITS
VEGETABLES — EXCEPT CORN, WHICH IS
A GRAIN
SELECTED FATS AND OILS, SUCH AS
COCONUT OIL, OLIVE OIL, AVOCADO
OIL, LARD, TALLOW, GHEE/BUTTER
MINIMALLY PROCESSED SWEETENERS,
INCLUDING RAW HONEY, MAPLE SYRUP,
COCONUT SUGAR, RAW STEVIA

BAN LIST
LEGUMES: BEANS, LENTILS, PEAS,
PEANUTS, ETC.
DAIRY: MILK, CHEESE, BUTTER, ICE
CREAM, YOGURT, ETC.
MOST COOKING OILS: VEGETABLE,
CANOLA, CORN, PEANUT, PALM, ETC.
GRAINS: CEREAL GRAINS, CORN,
WHEAT, QUINOA, RICE, PASTA, GRITS,
ETC.

WHAT'S THE DIFFERENCE

keto vs paleo

"The paleo diet is definitely more
liberal than the keto diet, because
you have more options, and you
can have more fruits and
vegetables"

Paleo - less strict on ratios

Atkins

LOW CARB DIET WITH 4 PHASES
PHASE 1 (INDUCTION)
PHASE 2 (BALANCING)
PHASE 3 (FINE-TUNING)
PHASE 4 (MAINTENANCE)

WHAT YOU CAN EAT
MEATS: BEEF, PORK, LAMB, CHICKEN, BACON AND OTHERS.
FATTY FISH AND SEAFOOD: SALMON, TROUT, SARDINES, ETC.
EGGS: THE HEALTHIEST EGGS ARE OMEGA-3 ENRICHED OR PASTURED.
LOW-CARB VEGETABLES: KALE, SPINACH, BROCCOLI, ASPARAGUS AND OTHERS.
FULL-FAT DAIRY: BUTTER, CHEESE, CREAM, FULL-FAT YOGURT.
NUTS AND SEEDS: ALMONDS, MACADAMIA NUTS, WALNUTS, SUNFLOWER SEEDS. ETC.
HEALTHY FATS: EXTRA VIRGIN OLIVE OIL, COCONUT OIL, AVOCADOS AND AVOCADO OIL.

BAN LIST
SUGAR: SOFT DRINKS, FRUIT JUICES, CAKES, CANDY, ICE CREAM, ETC.
GRAINS: WHEAT, SPELT, RYE, BARLEY, RICE.
VEGETABLE OILS: SOYBEAN OIL, CORN OIL, COTTONSEED OIL, CANOLA OIL AND A FEW OTHERS.
TRANS FATS: USUALLY FOUND IN PROCESSED FOODS WITH THE WORD "HYDROGENATED" ON THE INGREDIENTS LIST.
"DIET" AND "LOW-FAT" FOODS: THESE ARE USUALLY VERY HIGH IN SUGAR.
HIGH-CARB VEGETABLES: CARROTS, TURNIPS, ETC (INDUCTION ONLY).
HIGH-CARB FRUITS: BANANAS, APPLES, ORANGES, PEARS, GRAPES (INDUCTION ONLY).
STARCHES: POTATOES, SWEET POTATOES (INDUCTION ONLY).
LEGUMES: LENTILS, BEANS, CHICKPEAS, ETC. (INDUCTION ONLY).

I.F

INTERMITTENT FASTING IS NOT A DIET, IT'S A PATTERN OF EATING. IT'S A WAY OF SCHEDULING YOUR MEALS SO THAT YOU GET THE MOST OUT OF THEM. INTERMITTENT FASTING DOESN'T CHANGE WHAT YOU EAT, IT CHANGES WHEN YOU EAT.

12:12 METHOD
FAST FOR 12 HOURS A DAY AND EAT WITHIN A 12-HOUR WINDOW. IF YOU EAT YOUR LAST MEAL AT 7 P.M. AND HAVE BREAKFAST THE NEXT MORNING AT 7 A.M.,

20:4 METHOD
FAST FOR A FULL 20 HOURS AND ALLOW YOURSELF ONE FOUR-HOUR WINDOW TO EAT.

16:8 METHOD
EAT YOUR DAILY FOOD WITHIN AN 8-HOUR WINDOW AND FAST FOR THE REMAINING 16 HOURS.

5:2 METHOD
EAT WHATEVER YOU WANT FOR 5 DAYS OUT OF THE WEEK.

WHAT YOU CAN EAT
ANYTHING YOU WANT

BAN LIST
NOTHING

D.I.E...T

Juicing

ABSTAINING FROM EATING OTHER FOODS
AND ONLY DRINKING JUICE
USUALLY LIMITED TO A SHORT PERIOD OF
TIME – OFTEN BETWEEN THREE DAYS AND
ONE WEEK.

WHAT YOU CAN DRINK
SQUEEZED OR COLD PRESSED VEGE/FRUIT
JUICE

BAN LIST
NO ADDED SUGAR

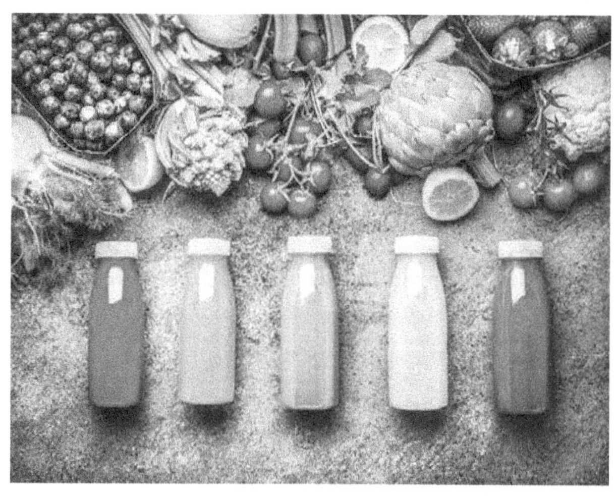

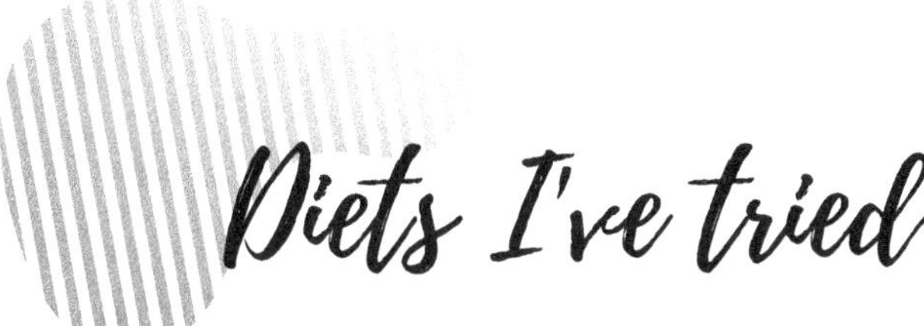

Diets I've tried

What I ate   **Why it didn't work**

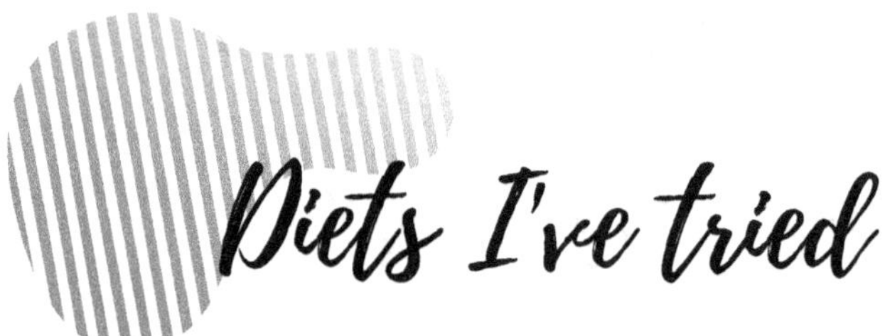

What I ate

Why it didn't work

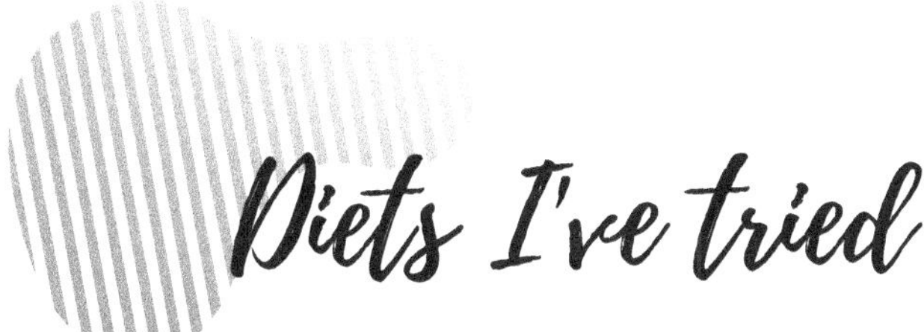

Diets I've tried

What I ate   Why it didn't work

EAT-ONLY-ONE-THING

aka the mono diet. As in you only eat 1 food item. The inspiration for this diet is Penn Jilette, the magician, who underwent a huge transformation. Take a look..

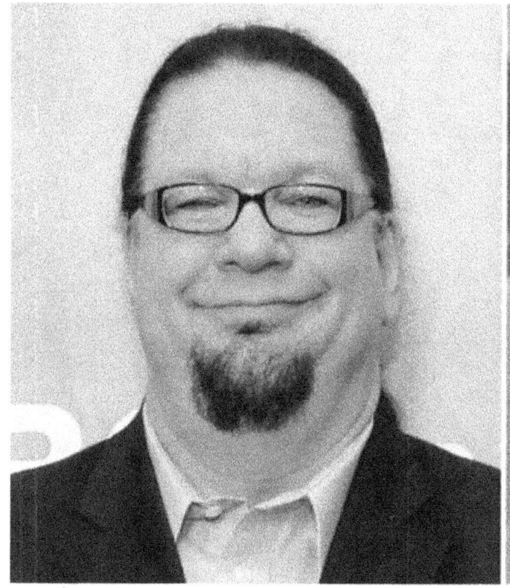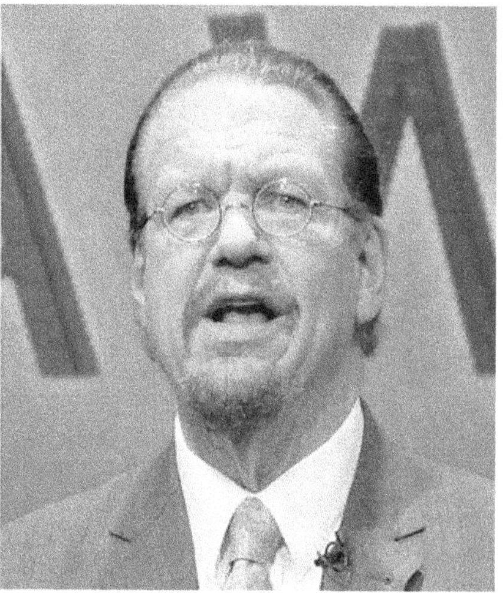

The principle behind this diet is to only eat one food, instead of eating all carbs or protein or only juicing. Eat only boiled potatoes for 2 weeks (with no added seasoning) to reset your body. Drink all the coffee / tea that you want, minus the sugar.

Understandably, this diet cannot be sustained on a long term basis but within the first 5 days, you see immediate results (flatter belly) and this serves to motivate and jumpstart the weight loss.

Variants of this include egg or fruit only diet.

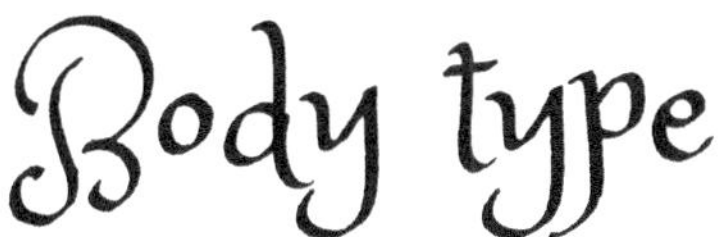

Body type

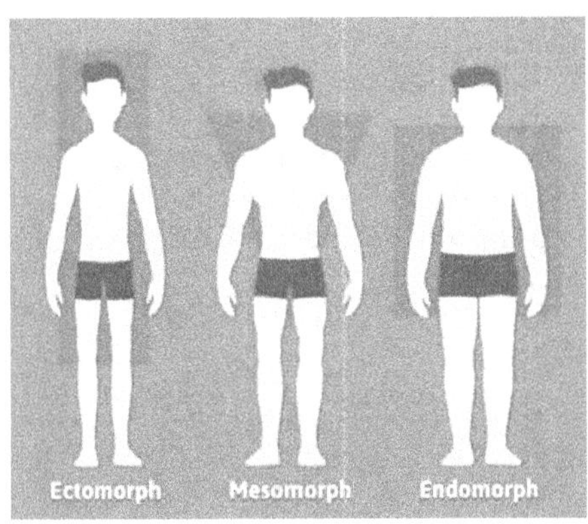

Why do some people lose weight so easily? Or worse, without even trying.

Why do others try one diet and get results?

I tried the same diet, but I did not lose weight as much as him/her. Why is that?

Many factors. Age, body type, metabolism, gut health…to name a few. You just haven't found a way of eating (diet) that suits your body.

ECTOMORPH

Fashion models have ectomorph bodies.
Put down this book. Why do you need to lose weight? Carbs...you need more carbs!

2 palms of protein dense foods at each meal;
2 fists of vegetables at each meal;
3 cupped handfuls of carb dense foods at each meal;
1 thumb of fat dense foods at each meal.

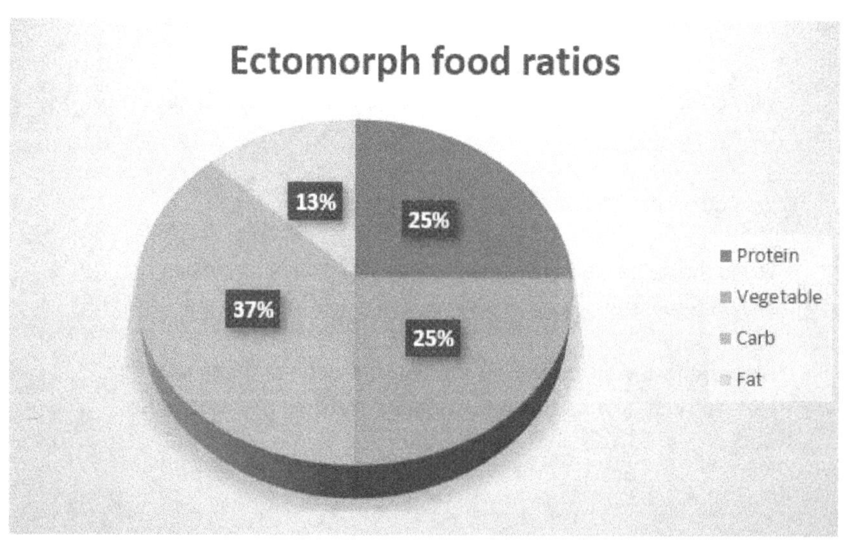

MESOMORPH

Eat balanced vegs, proteins and carbs
2 palms of protein dense foods
at each meal;
2 fists of vegetables at each
meal;
2 cupped handfuls of carb dense
foods at each meal;
2 thumb of fat dense foods
at each meal.

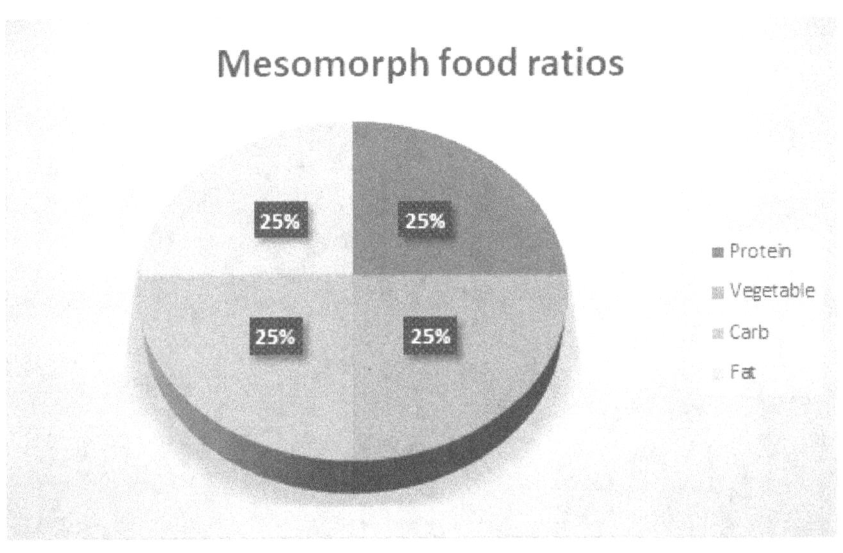

ENDOMORPH

Mesomorphs tend to turn into endos when they get older.

**Eat food in these ratios
2 palms of protein dense foods
at each meal;
2 fists of vegetables at each
meal;
1 cupped handful of carb dense
foods at each meal;
3 thumbs of fat dense foods
at each meal.**

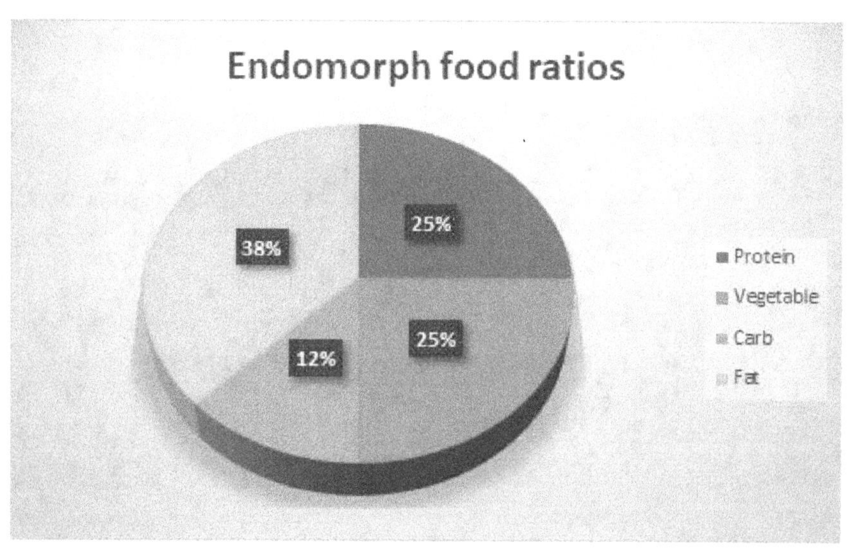

How to tell IS IT WORKING?

When should you stop the diet?

* when your energy runs low
* when you frequently get sick (flu, cough...)
* dizziness, migraine, joint pain, bloating, constipation
* no longer enjoy meals
* difficulty getting up from bed
* fluctuating weight (+ then -)
* lost meaning of life :)

When should you NOT stop the diet?

* no weight loss
* weight gain
* people making fun of you
* clothes feeling looser

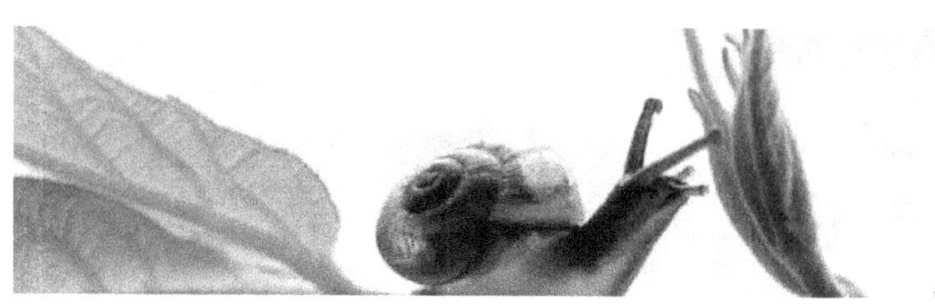

Slow down

What it means is

...get the phone out of your face, no reading or cute kitty videos while eating

...food in mouth, chew chew chew chew chew, don't talk in between chews, chew chew chew, swallow

...scoop up next portion (by that I mean, there should be no portion of food in your spoon waiting while you chew)

...every now and then, take a sip of water

...if your stomach says full, then stop even if there's still food on the plate

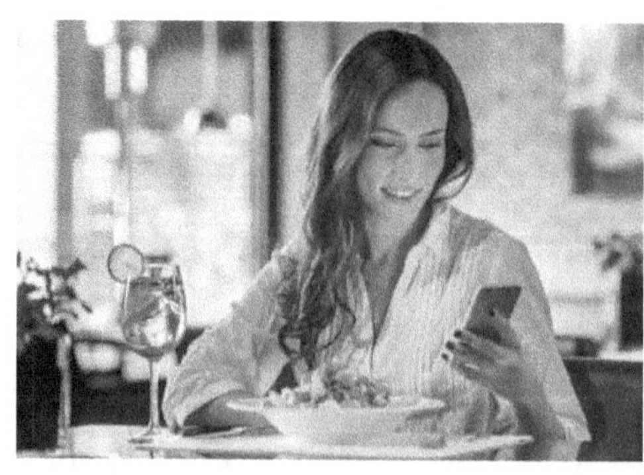

DON'T QUIT

The problem with diets are sustainability. Sure you can start the next new fancy schmancy diet at the start of the New Year. You buy a shitload of healthy food, clear the fridge etc, follow the diet plan, log your meals....for the first 2 weeks.

And then... you step on the scale (after taking a number 2 and removing every article of clothing; because every gram counts!).

After all that restraint and suffering, you lost a grand total of 500 grams.

Wait, what?!

It's easy to give up when you don't see immediate results. And you expected to see significant weight loss after a short period of time.

Wake up.

You've been eating wrong and gaining the weight for years. Your body needs time to reset.

Give yourself time.

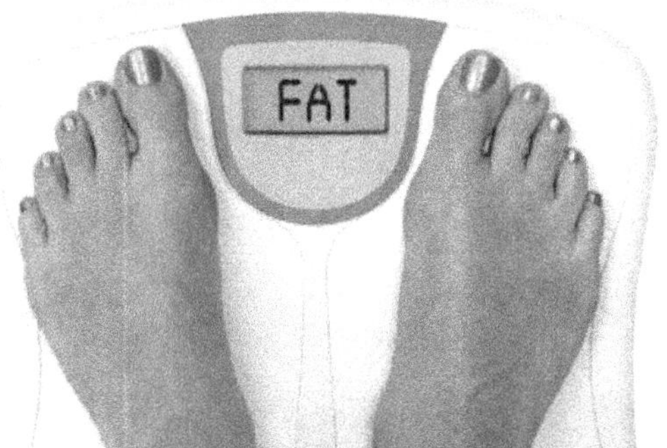

pavlovian response

1. DOG SALIVATES ON SEEING FOOD
2. BELL RINGS, DOG HAS NO RESPONSE
3. DOG SALIVATES WHEN SEEING FOOD, BELL IS RUNG
4. DOG SALIVATES WHEN BELL IS RUNG

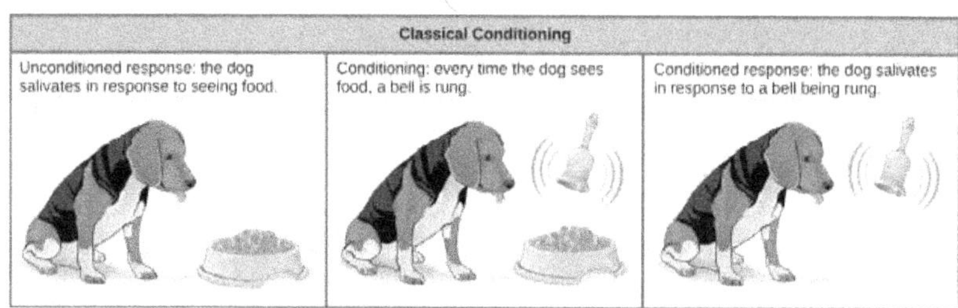

THE THEORY IS CLASSICAL CONDITIONING.
PEOPLE ASSOCIATE TWO STIMULI IN THEIR MINDS AND
REACT TO ONE OF THEM AS THOUGH IT WAS THE OTHER.

pavlovian response

LET'S LEARN FROM A DOG

YOU HAVE TURKEY FOR THANKSGIVING. IT IS A TIME FOR FAMILY AND YOU ASSOCIATE TURKEY WITH HAPPY MEMORIES. SO WHEN YOU HAVE TURKEY OUT OF SEASON, YOU WILL HAVE FOND MEMORIES AND FEEL HAPPY WHILE EATING TURKEY.

SAME REASON SOME OF US LOVE CANDY AND SWEETS. IT'S A THROWBACK FROM CHILDHOOD, BACK WHEN TIMES WERE SIMPLE AND YOU WERE CAREFREE. HAVING A PIECE OF CANDY EQUATES TO REMINISCING YOUR CHILDHOOD.

NOW LET'S FLIP THE COIN. YOU WERE DRINKING MILK TEA WHEN YOUR BOYFRIEND/GIRLFRIEND BREAKS UP WITH YOU. IT IS A TRAUMATIC EXPERIENCE. CHANCES ARE YOU WILL REFRAIN FROM DRINKING MILK TEA WHEN YOU CAN AVOID IT AS YOU ASSOCIATE IT WITH THE EXPERIENCE OF BREAKING UP. JUST AS YOU WOULD AVOID CERTAIN PLACES YOU USED TO VISIT AS A COUPLE TOGETHER.

USE THIS PAVLOVIAN RESPONSE TO HELP YOU LOSE WEIGHT. GOT A SWEET TOOTH HABIT YOU JUST CAN'T BREAK? WHILE EATING YOUR FAVORITE INDULGENCE, CALL UP A BAD MEMORY. IMMERSE YOURSELF IN THAT MEMORY. YES, YOUR BRAIN CAN BE EASILY FOOLED IF YOU KNOW HOW. DO IT MULTIPLE TIMES UNTIL THE SIGHT OF THE FOOD CAUSES THE MEMORY TO SURFACE.

MIND OVER MATTER

HUNGRY IMMIGRANT MENTALITY

Have you ever looked at old childhood pictures and sigh?
I used to be so thin, you'd lament.

So what has changed? Besides the age factor which contributes to your metabolism, when you were a child or teenager or a university student, you had an allowance. You lived under the roof of your parents and your meals depended on them. When you wanted ice cream for dessert, it wasn't always a YES. Sometimes you had to clean your room beforehand or take out the garbage. That is a big factor to weight gain. There was an element of CONTROL, enforced by your parents.

Once you started earning your own salary, your appetite and weight goes off the roof. You'd see that muffin that you like, and purchase it without much thought. After all, you deserve it after a grueling day at the office.

Now I'd like you to reminisce. When you were facing exams or was stressed out, did you binge eat? You had other ways to cope, right? It is only during adulthood that majority choose food as comfort because to be honest, most of us are stuck in the office and there's simply no other way to alleviate stress. Food is always within easy reach. When you were young, you could go outdoors, shoot some baskets, go window shopping and come back fresh.

So, the simple solution to this is simply to limit yourself. Have a hungry immigrant mentality, where you only have a certain amount of money for food daily or weekly. Doesn't matter whether you eat out or cook. You either plan your meals or starve before the week or day is over. This method not only lightens your body but saves you extra money in the long run also.

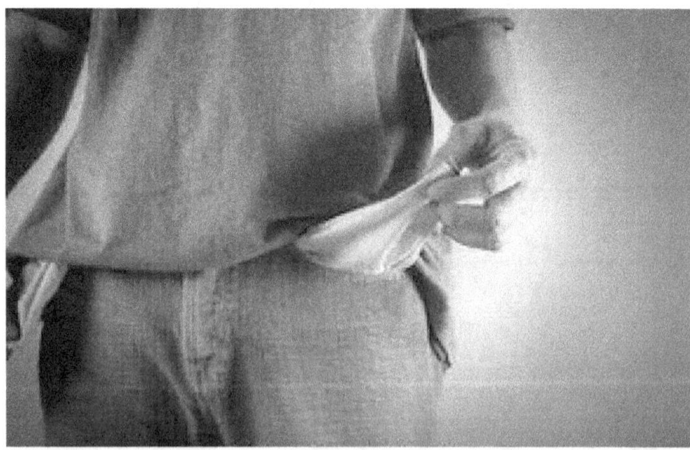

STOP SELF DELUSIONS

Selfie on phones feed your self delusion. It applies filters to your complexion, gives you a sharper jawline, removes your double chin...

That's not what you look like in real life. As time goes by, you start to believe the lie. You forget that the beauty filter was set to maximum.

And when you turn it off, you get the shock of your life.

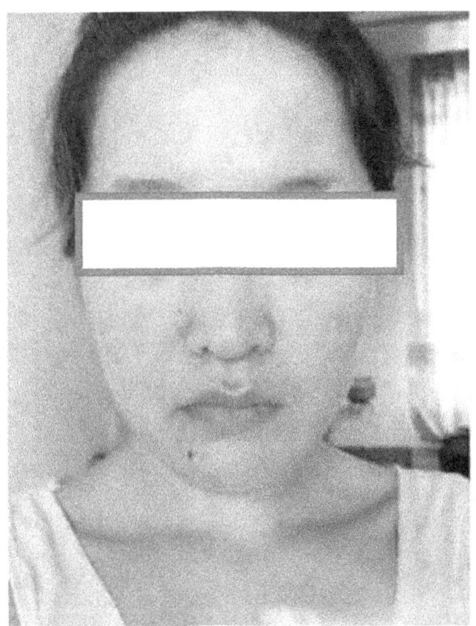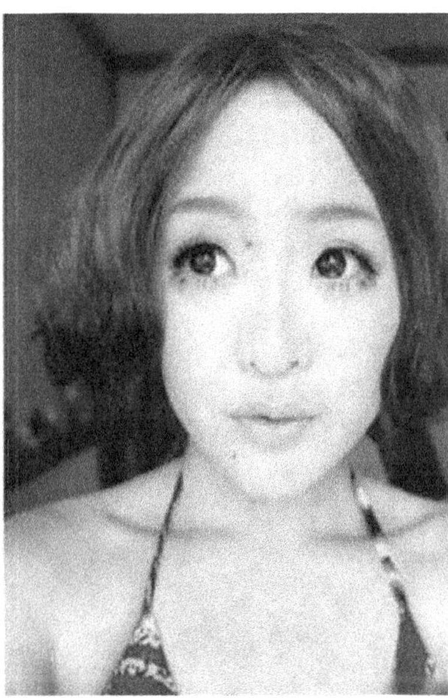

TOXIC PEOPLE

You are what you eat. That is a very frightening thought. If this were true, most of us would be doughnut shaped.

The average adult spends 8 hours a day working, of which they are granted one hour of lunchtime. That's equivalent to 5 hours a week, 104 hours a year. Some people dine alone but most have a group of lunch friends with whom to eat with.

One word of advice. Choose your lunch mates wisely. Normally the decision on where or what to eat lies in majority. And a majority of people don't make wise or healthy decisions. You would generally go with the flow in order not to be labeled an outcast. But what if you were on a healthy eating plan? What if you chose to bring home cooked food?

Some lunch mates sneer or try to discourage you by criticizing that they see no difference in your weight even though you were eating healthy. Even the simplest remark sting if it came from a friend. You'd feel bad and rejoin the crowd. Others tempt you with their food to test your willpower.

My advice, stay firm and true to yourself. Listen to your inner voice, you own your body, you have to deal with the consequences of eating unhealthy food for a long period of time. If necessary, eat alone and schedule a once weekly lunchtime with those colleagues in order to catch up.

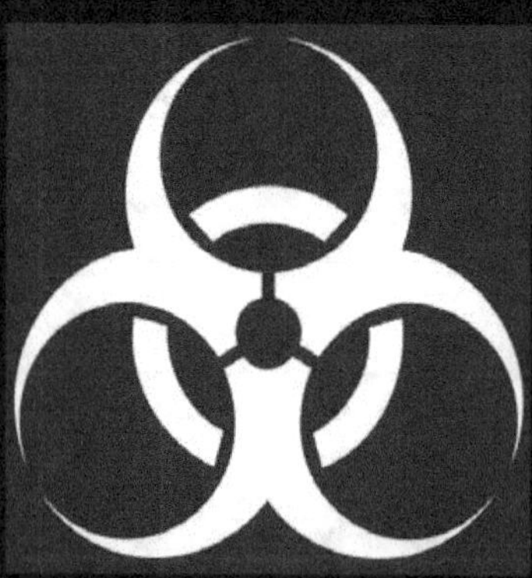

MAKE A BUDGET

Limit your meal budget to $20 a day. That means

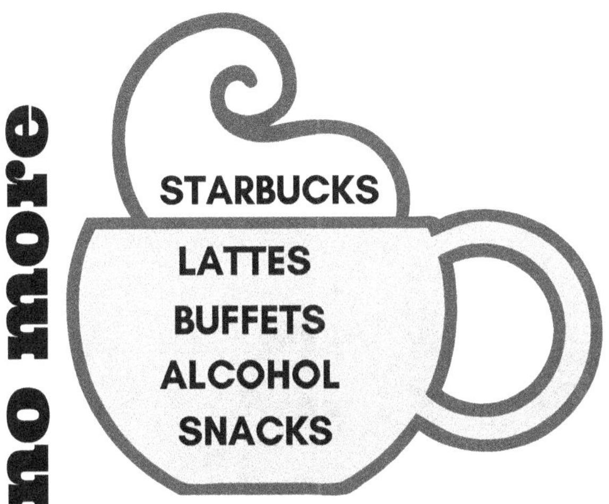

Stretch your dollar. See how far you can go.
The cheapest & healthiest option is to prepare your own meals.

ONE POT RECIPES

When you cook at home, you control the portions, the spices, the salt, sugar etc

After a stressful day in the office, the simple routine of cooking takes your mind off things.

The crock pot and pressure cooker are your new BFFs. Dump your food inside, set and forget.

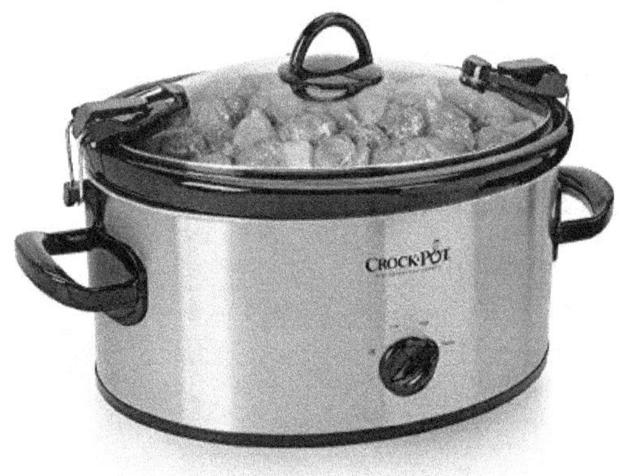

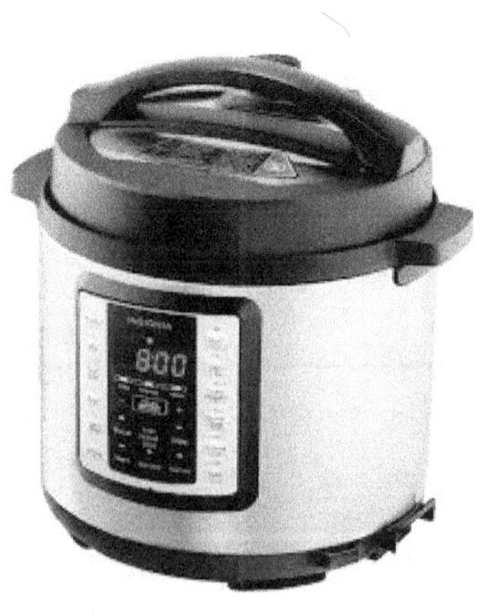

RECIPE 1

Have at least 3 no brainer fallback one pot recipes. The ingredients must have a long shelf life and are always available in your fridge.

Example:

1.
2.
3.

Mushroom pasta
Chicken noodle soup
Potato salad / omelette

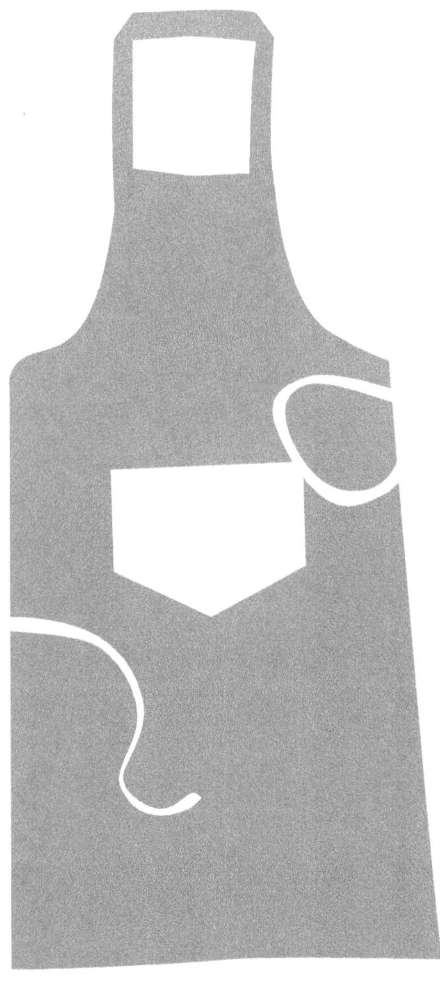

RECIPE 2

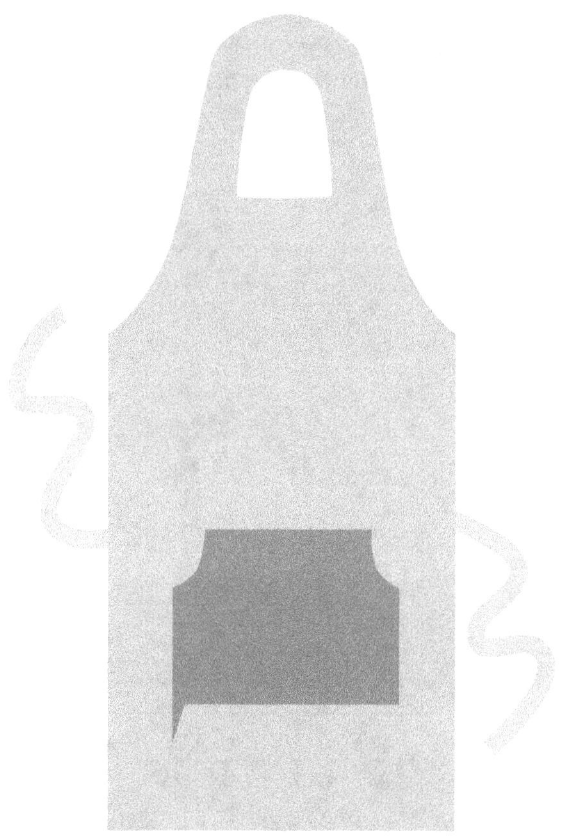

RECIPE 3

COOL RECIPES

Healthy food is expensive. It takes longer to make.
It's more convenient to reach for fast food or eat out. When you eat out, you lose control of what gets added to your food. If you observe a famous iced tea being made in local restaurants, you'd shudder at the amount of sugar they use. No wonder the tea tasted so delicious!

The cheapest and fastest way for weight loss is to prepare your own food. Don't put your health in the hands of others.

OAT in JAR is one of my fave recipes because I am lazy and these can be made in a batch. When I get hunger pangs, I just reach for a jar.

RECIPE

Oat in Jar!

1. ONE SERVING OF EAT INTO A GLASS JAR
2. FILL UP JAR UNTIL OAT IS COVERED WITH ANY MILK OF YOUR DESIRE
3. ADD TOPPING (IDEAS BELOW)
4. PUT THE LID ON AND STORE IN FRIDGE
MAKE A BATCH OF 5 JARS AND YOU'RE SET FOR THE WEEK

TOPPING IDEAS

+ almond / any nut!
+ peanut butter
+ chia seed
+ ginger powder
+ any fruit
+ chocolate

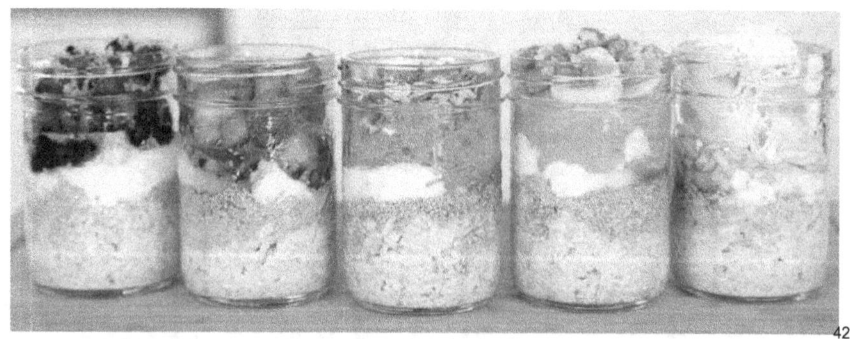

Energy Bar

GOOD FOR POO
GOOD FOR HEART
CONVENIENT TO GRAB FOR QUICK ENERGY BOOST
CHEWY AND LOOKS LIKE HAMSTER FOOD

AVOID YOGHURT BARS SOLD IN MARTS

I ONLY GO FOR CARMAN'S (THIS IS NOT AN
INFOMERCIAL, IT JUST GIVES ME NICE POO)

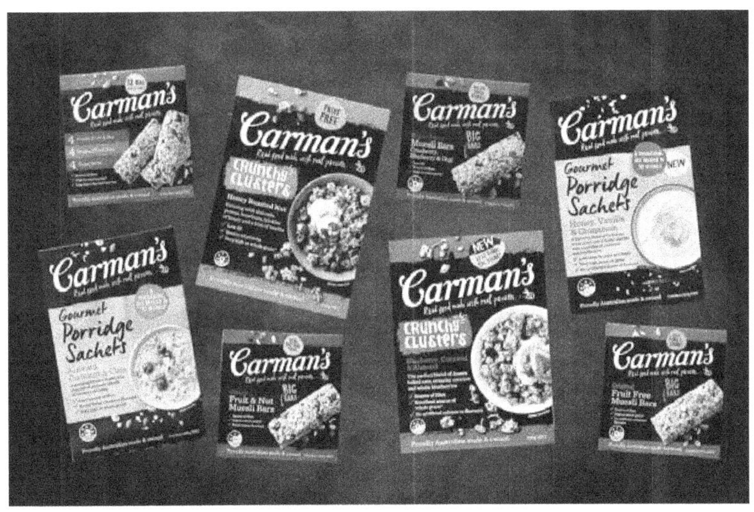

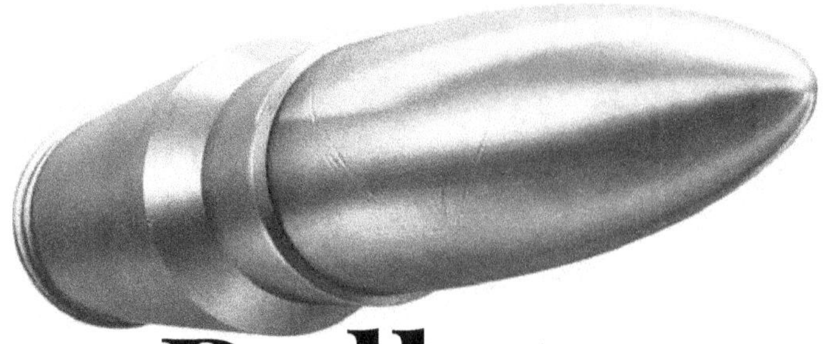

Bulletproof Coffee

COFFEE + BUTTER + MCT OIL / COCONUT OIL

Why it's good for you

* clearer mind
* caffeine is released slowly through the body (to prevent caffeine crash)
* coffee + *fat = high energy
* weight loss

*Fat is an essential part of almost every physiologic function in our body, particularly when it comes to optimal brain function

EXORCISE THE HOME

STEP 1

REMOVE ALL EDIBLE ITEMS FROM ALL ROOMS
EXCEPT THE KITCHEN

STEP 2

PLACE A BOTTLE OF DRINKABLE WATER IN EVERY
ROOM INCLUDING THE KITCHEN

STEP 3

GOTO KITCHEN.
DISPOSE OF THE FOLLOWING
* EXPIRED FOOD
* PROCESSED FOOD
* SUGARED DRINKS

STEP 4

OPEN YOUR FRIDGE
REPEAT STEP 3

STEP 5

GOTO THE NEAREST FRESH FOOD MART
BUY THE FOLLOWING
* FRESH VEG
* LOTS OF FRUIT
* SEA SALT
* WHOLE MEAT (NOTHING MINCED)
* YOGHURT / PROBIOTIC
(IF YOU CAN TOLERATE IT)
* NUTS
* OAT
* EGGS
* GREEN TEA

h2o

I hate water.
It's plain, it's clear, it's tasteless.
I   drank water so infrequently my grandma used to say my intestines would stick together (technically they are!). I tried to meet my daily intake through bowls and bowls of soup, coffee and fruits.
Water holds benefits that cannot be ignored.
Think of it as lubricant for your internals since 70% of your body consists of water. When we get sick, mothers and friends tell us to REST and DRINK MORE WATER.
So in order to 'trick' myself to drink more water, I have to come up with creative ways to flavor my water.

Since fruit is so healthy, a popular way is to have fruit infused water. Basically you dump your choice of fruit into the water, let it infuse, and then drink away.

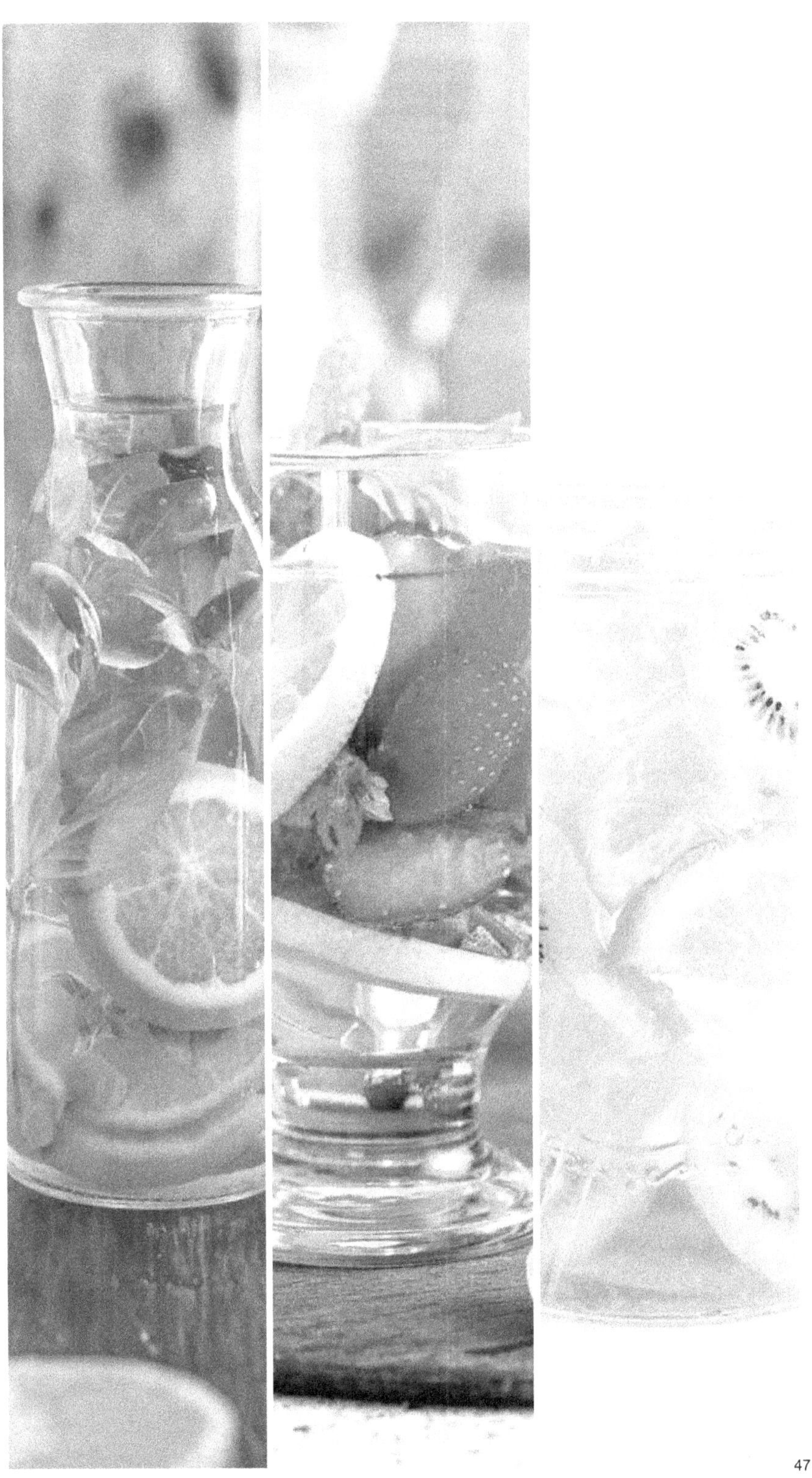

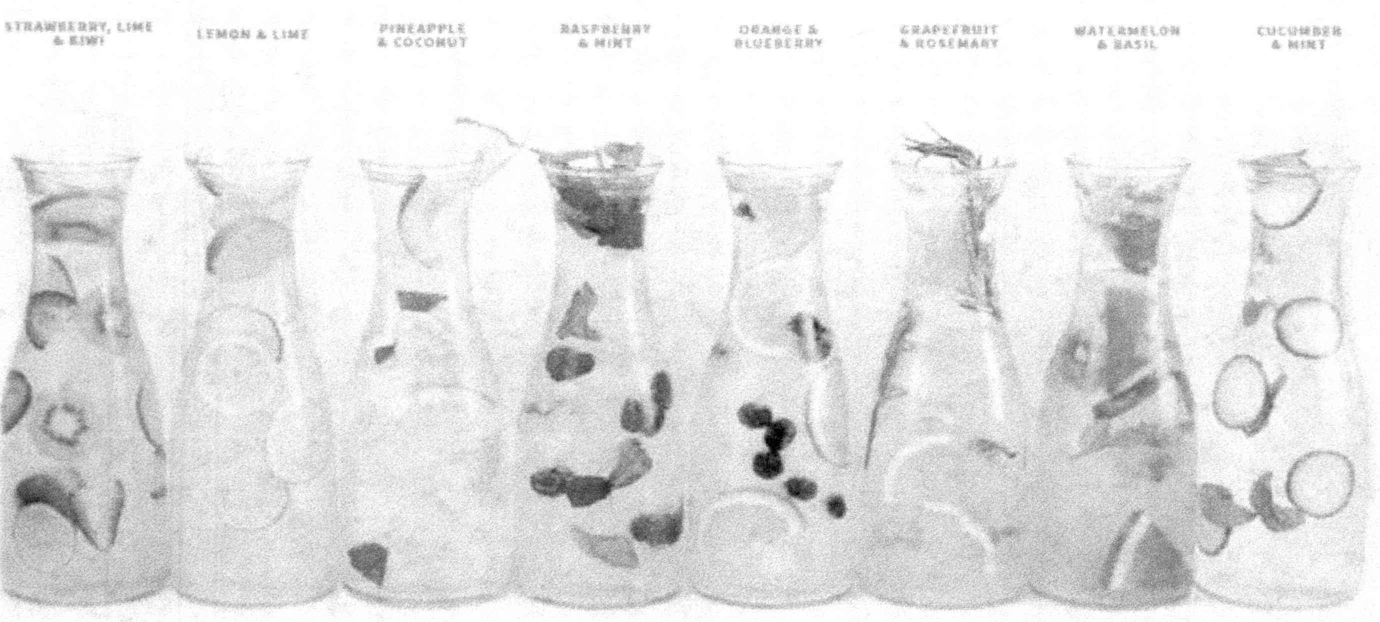

STRAWBERRY, LIME & KIWI
LEMON & LIME
PINEAPPLE & COCONUT
RASPBERRY & MINT
ORANGE & BLUEBERRY
GRAPEFRUIT & ROSEMARY
WATERMELON & BASIL
CUCUMBER & MINT

h2O

the many flavors of water

If you live in a country where the tap water is not drinkable, avoid reverse osmosis water (RO). Only go for mineral water.

Once a day, add a dash of sea salt (I know, it tastes weird)
Sea salt gives you
* vitamins and minerals
* clearer skin
* good digestion

Please don't confuse regular table salt with sea salt.

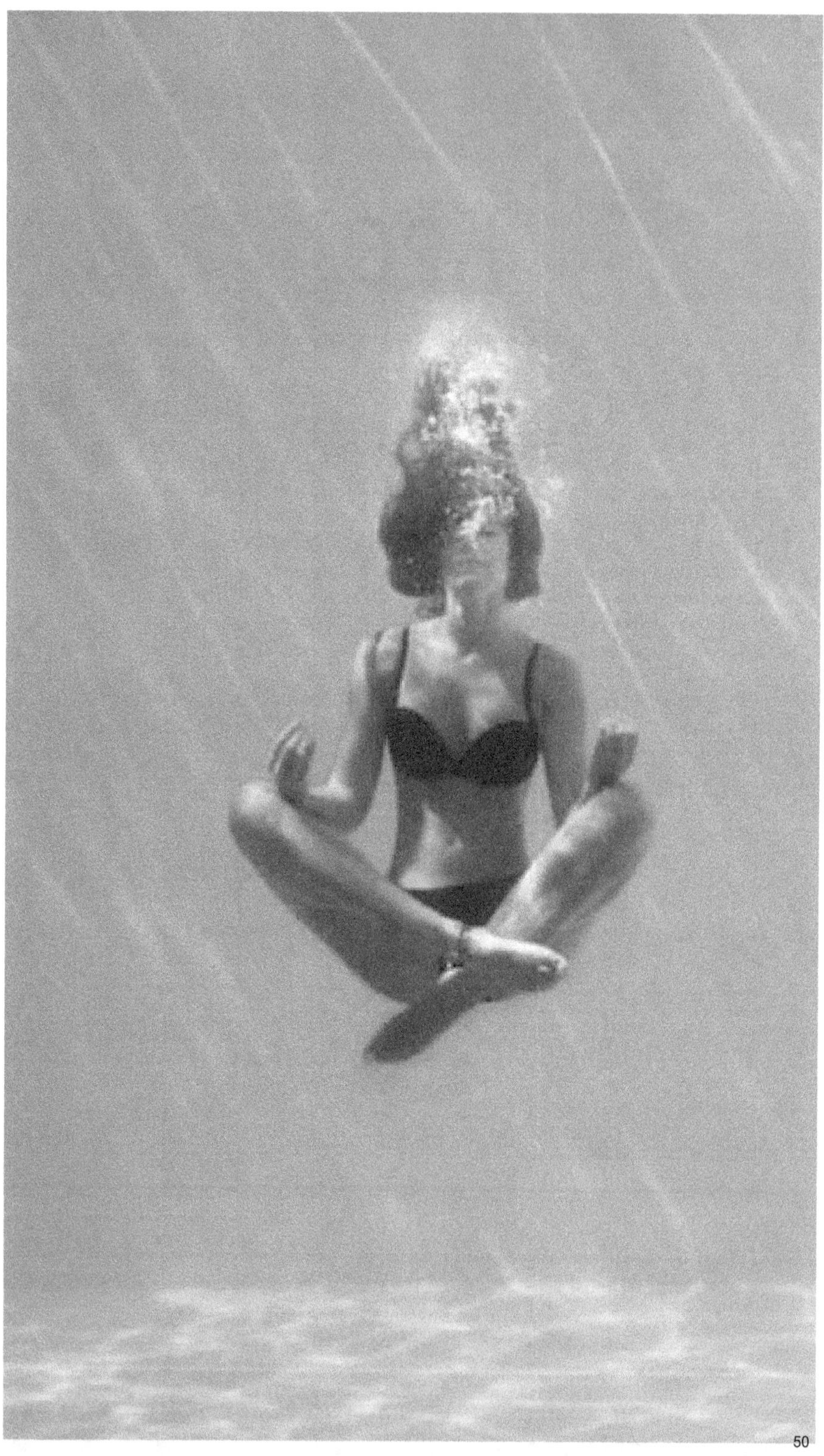

FRUIT MYTHS

MYTH #1
must be eaten on empty stomach

FACT: Eat them anytime. Nutritional value remain the same. But if you eat them on an empty stomach, you feel full faster

MYTH #2
fruit juice = whole fruit

FACT: fruit juice may contain added sugars and lacks fibre. If you are really lazy to chew, get cold pressed juice

MYTH #3
fruit has sugar. sugar is bad.

FACT: fruit contain natural sugar sucrose, fructose and glucose
Health risks come from free sugars, not natural sugar

Cold-pressed juices are made from special machines that crush and press the fruits and veggies to extract the juice. There is no spinning and blades involved.
Cold pressed juicers are very effective in retaining nutrients. The juice also lasts for more days than regular juice and is the go-to drink for a cleanse.

MODERATION
IS THE KEY

apple cider

"Adding 1 or 2 tablespoons of apple cider vinegar to your diet can help you lose weight. It can also reduce your body fat percentage, make you lose belly fat and decrease your blood triglycerides. This is one of a few human studies that have investigated vinegar's effects on weight loss."

Apple cider in its raw form is horrible to taste.
If Satan were in a bad mood and perspiring, this would be the taste of his sweat.
Since the concoction helps you lose weight, we shall have to tolerate it by finding ways to neutralize its foul taste.

Things you can combine ACV with:

apple cider
+ honey
+ tea
+ avocado
egg salad
+ ginger lemon

What's guaranteed, this will be your expression once you consume it.

WORKOUT FOR BEGINNERS

If you were a newbie, working out (anywhere!) can be daunting. Your mind is traitorous and can think up a million excuses for you NOT to get started.

The important point is simply to GET STARTED.
GET OFF THE COUCH. If you really have to watch that TV drama, watch it while working out.

You're afraid you'd look silly. You're not sure which exercises to do. Are you doing it correctly? Is my bone supposed to crack so loudly?

The best workouts are workouts that require no equipment, but your own bodyweight. You can workout anytime, anywhere. Here are a few beginner exercises to help get you back into the game.

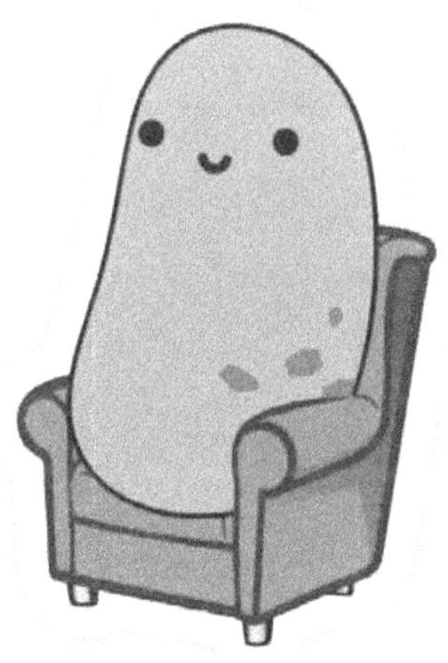

WORKOUT FOR BEGINNERS

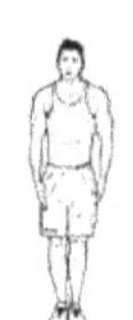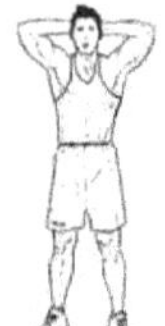

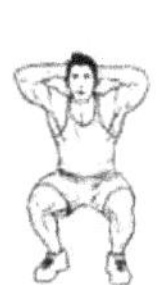

Jumping Jacks / Star Jumps
40 secs

Bodyweight Squat
2 sets / 8 reps

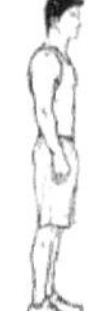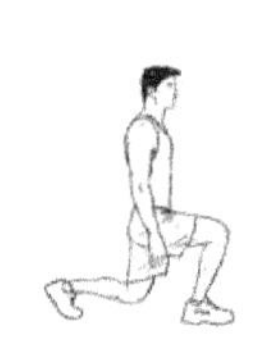

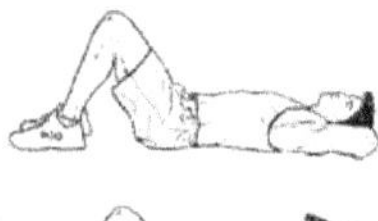
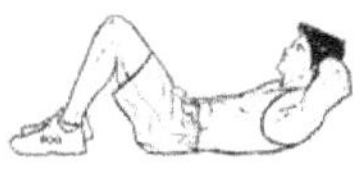

Bodyweight Walking Lunge
2 sets / 8 reps

Crunches
2 sets / 15 reps

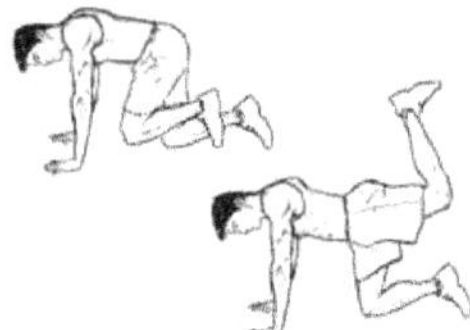

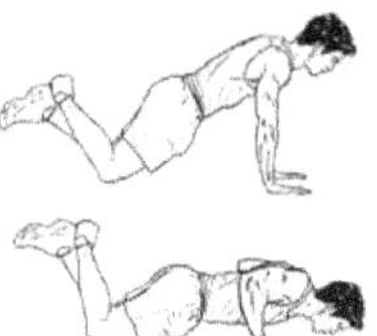

Donkey Kicks
2 sets / 8 reps

Modified / Knee Push-up
2 sets

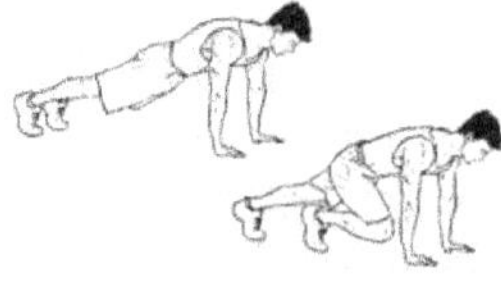
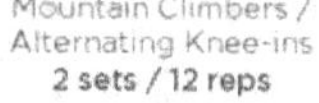

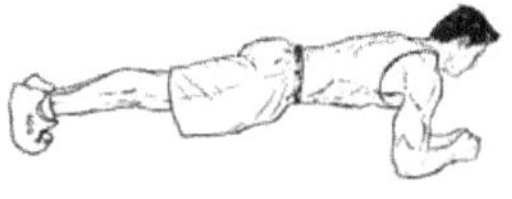

Mountain Climbers /
Alternating Knee-ins
2 sets / 12 reps

Plank
20 secs

Get a new workout everyday
www.darebee.com

WORKOUT
EVERYWHERE

Walk the dog / cat / hamster / snake / iguana / the kid

Park far from everywhere

If you work on the 10th floor, get off at 6th

Set a timer to get away from your desk every half hour

Do not have groceries delivered

Aim to elevate your heartbeat at least once a day

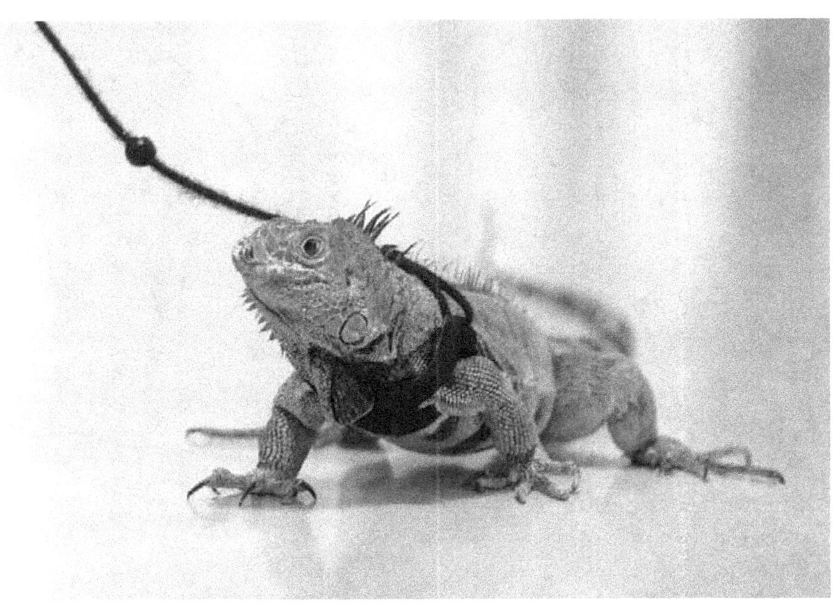

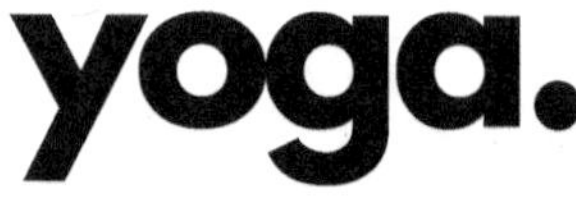

yoga.

FOR FEMINISTS

Nothing like a sun salutation to kickstart your morning. Yoga promotes proper breathing, good joint health, bloodflow and it's meditation for your soul. If you're like me and too cheapskate or shy to join a local class (where a teacher can correct and torture you!), then follow along to a good Youtube video.

Mark off these sessions on your phone to turn it into a habit. Use the template at the end of this book.

I recommend BOHO Beautiful and Adrienne on youtube.

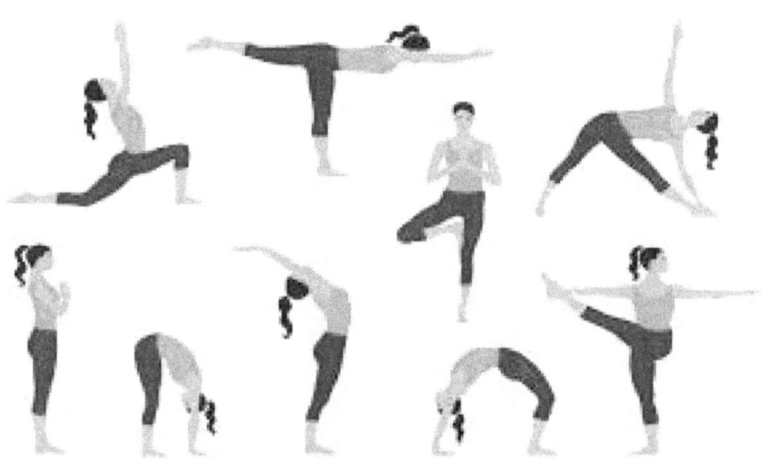

animal flow

Yoga too gentle for you? Go back to basics with functional movement or animal flow. These movement cover your whole body range of motion and forces your muscles to function as a group (instead of individually like most weight training).

If functional movement is too boring to you, try animal flow. Here's a hint, you enjoyed animal movement when you were a kid.

Ground based movement + pick a 4 legged animal = animal flow

If you still cannot imagine animal flow, remember SAMARA from the Ring?

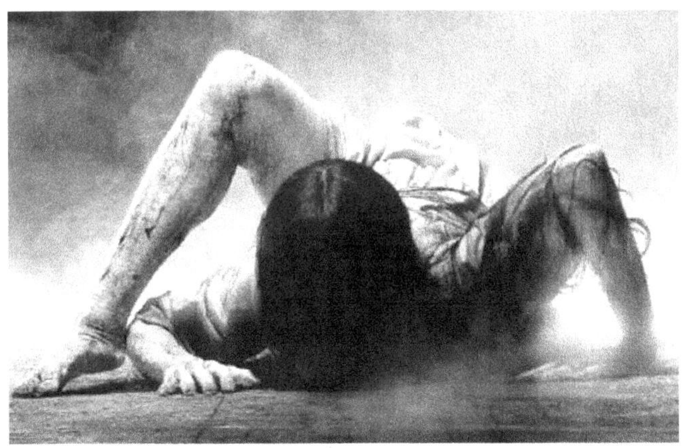

the ultitttet tittl flot MASTER

mindset

Your mind is an SOB. If you let it control you, it's going to tell you that you need a cheat day. "Today was a bad day" it whispers, "have a doughnut, you deserve it".
or
"Job well done! Let's order a pizza to celebrate!"

What an asshole, right?

"You'll never lose weight, what's the point of trying?"

How long can you resist yourself?

The only way to change your mind (literally!), is to change your mindset. Take rein of your life. Stop justifying certain foods, stop doubting yourself. Sure the mind will bitch and moan about missing its daily sugar fix, it is a habit that you've let it get away with for years.

And the biggest argument you can give your treacherous mind is by weighing yourself everyday. When your weight remains stubbornly static or worse increases, the seeds of doubt are planted. And the mind rationalizes that yours is a fruitless endeavor.

When you've showed your mind who's boss, you'd be surprised of how strong you actually are. And when you lose the extra weight, your mind will thank you for it. No more sugar crash, no more carb-induced fuzziness.

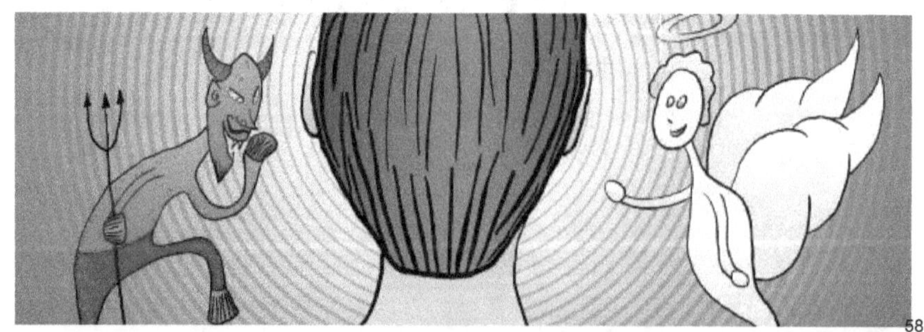

Compensating

Weight gain doesn't happen overnight. You don't go to sleep on Monday weighing 50kg and wake up Tuesday weighing 75kg.

It creeps up on you over time. You blink and 10 years have passed and you have gained 25 kg. WTF. How did you not notice it?

Because the pounds sneak in. It starts with the collar or waist pants getting tighter. And you shrug it off thinking that your clothes shrank in the dryer. So you buy new clothes, maybe a size or two bigger.

You step on the scale and you see you've gained a kilogram. It's the holidays, you can justify the weight gain. But it never comes off and the weight starts to pile on.

What matters is your response to these changes to your body. Do you procrastinate, or do something about it? Just like your school assignment, the longer you put it off, the more difficult it is to complete.

I used to be 65kg and hated my weight, and now I'm 72kg and wished I was still 65 kg.

So what are you waiting for?

Take action TODAY.

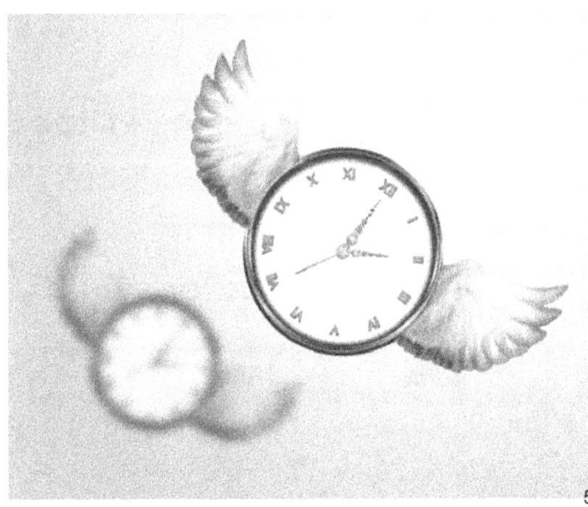

GEARS & TRACKERS

There's an important saying. You cannot improve what you cannot measure.

You say you're not sleeping well. Is that so? How long did you sleep? How many hours of light and deep sleep? Do you go to bed the same time every day?

You can't seem to lose weight. How many steps do you walk a day? Are you sedentary or lightly active or active? What is your average walking speed?

Did you work out today? What did you do? How long? What's the intensity? What was your heart rate?

We are lucky we live in an age where technology can be used to aid weight loss. They track your habits and now are even smart enough to give suggestions and remind you (just like a nagging mom!).

Data does not lie. Track your activity, analyse and tune them according to your needs.

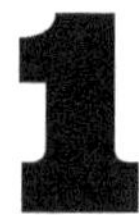

pedometer

Track your steps. Have a daily goal. See trends. Do you slack off more during the weekends?

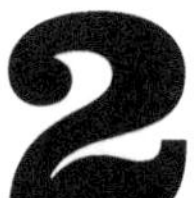

pedometer + heart rate

Same thing. With heart rate detection. Are you in cardio/fat loss zone?

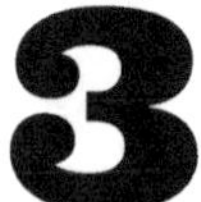

pedometer + blood pressure

The BP measurement is fake. Ignore. If you really must measure your BP, get the medical kind.

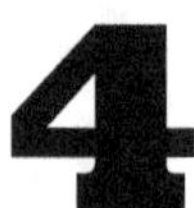

pedometer + GPS

Draws a nice path on a map of where you've been. Ideal if you jog /hike

gamify it

Make eating a game. Not a game of more, but a game of less. If you dine with friends, never let your order be the most expensive. Never let your food be more than the one next to you. Never be the last to finish eating.

If you have a fit friend, emulate what they eat. They must be doing something right. If he goes to the gym twice a week, you go thrice a week.

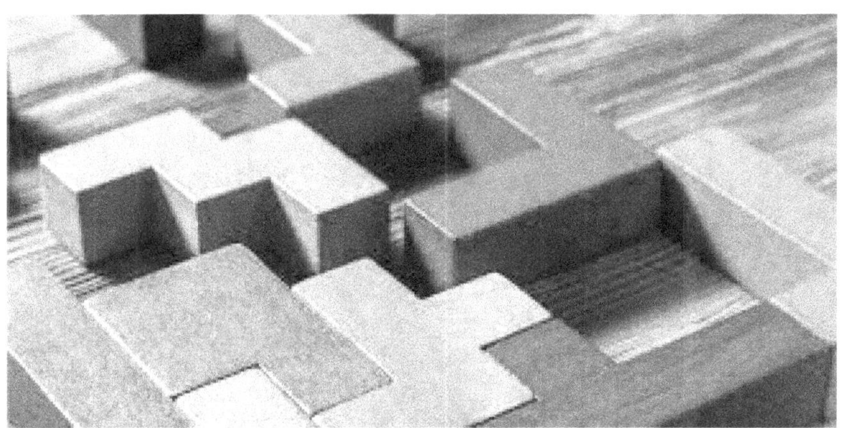

Good luck

THE AIM OF THIS BOOK IS TO PROVIDE YOU WITH IDEAS
(SOME OLD SOME NEW) ON YOUR WEIGHT LOSS JOURNEY.
A BOOK CAN ONLY SPOON FEED YOU INFORMATION AND
MOTIVATE YOU. BUT IT IS YOU ALONE WHO MUST TAKE
THE FIRST STEP.

I WISH YOU GOOD LUCK IN YOUR ADVENTURE.

KRISTINA ARCHER

Printable Templates

WHY YOU NEED THEM
* INSPIRATION
* MOTIVATION
* PROGRESS TRACKER
* ACCOUNTABILITY
* NO CHEAT

USE THE TEMPLATES BELOW AND PRINT MULTIPLE COPIES
AS NEEDED

CHEAT DAY tracker

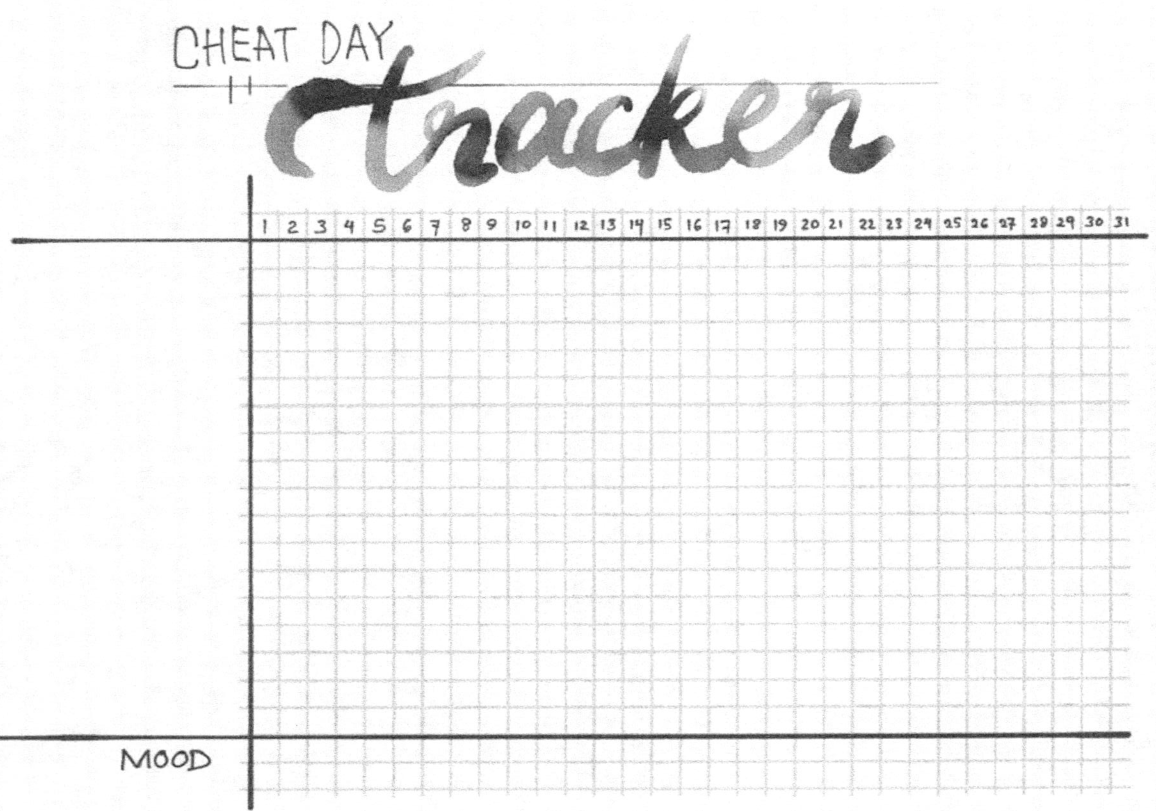

	MONDAY	TUESDAY	WEDNESDAY	THURSDAY	FRIDAY	SATURDAY	SUNDAY
BREAKFAST							
LUNCH							
SNACKS							
DINNER							
WORKOUT							

recipe card

NAME	INGREDIENTS

SERVES

TIME TO PREPARE

DIRECTIONS

TIME TO COOK

COOKING TEMP

TOOLS & UTENSILS

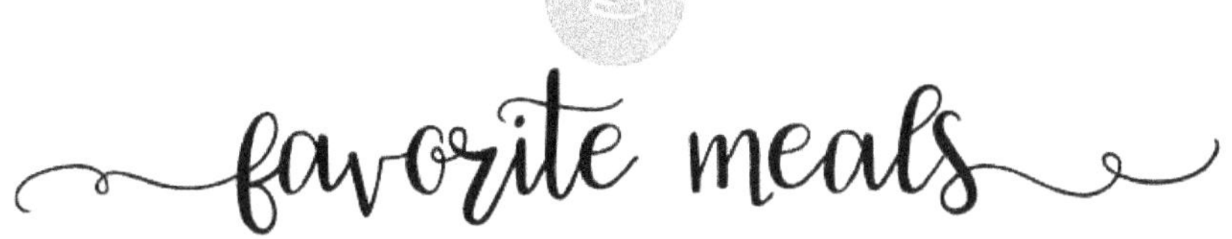

favorite meals

BREAKFAST

LUNCH

DINNER

DESSERTS

WEEKLY FITNESS *journal*

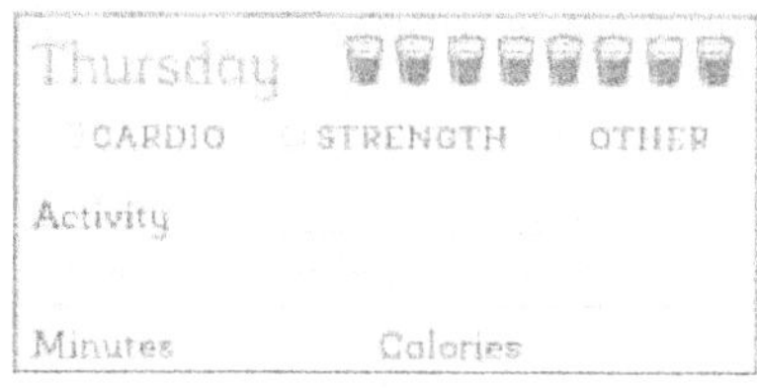

THIS WEEK'S GOALS

Sunday
CARDIO · STRENGTH · OTHER
Activity
Minutes · Calories

Monday
CARDIO · STRENGTH · OTHER
Activity
Minutes · Calories

Tuesday
CARDIO · STRENGTH · OTHER
Activity
Minutes · Calories

Wednesday
CARDIO · STRENGTH · OTHER
Activity
Minutes · Calories

Thursday
CARDIO · STRENGTH · OTHER
Activity
Minutes · Calories

Friday
CARDIO · STRENGTH · OTHER
Activity
Minutes · Calories

Saturday
CARDIO · STRENGTH · OTHER
Activity
Minutes · Calories

This Week's Check-In

Weight

Pounds Lost

meal planner